Alzheimer's

How to care, cope and prevent Alzheimer's

diseases.

Juliet Heffner

ISBN 10: 1722310413:
ISBN-13: 978-1722310417

CONTENTS

This page was intentionally left blank

CHAPTER ONE

Identifying the early symptoms of Alzheimer's disease

Alzheimer's disease is an illness that affects the mental health of its victims. It destroys the brain's capacity to function optimally. Studies show that people who smoke are 45% prone to Alzheimer's diseases. Recent statistics show an increasing number of Alzheimer's patient every year with people 60years and above taking a lion share of the menace. A study in July 2008 of Alzheimer and vascular dementia shows that 25.4% of the participants or 5367 people diagnosed with dementia an average of 23 years later. Of the patients with dementia 1136 were diagnosed with Alzheimer's diseases and 416 were vascular dementia

Alzheimer's diseases affect the mind and personality of the victim and slowly destroy their happiness. At the moments Alzheimer's diseases have no cure, but there are various drugs developed by scientists to delay the rapid progression of the dreaded. At the moment, early diagnosis of the disease is the best method of managing the ailment. Now what are the early symptoms of Alzheimer's diseases

Memory loss

Alzheimer's disease has the capacity to affect short-term memory of its patient, if you or anyone around you is having trouble with short-term memory loss that is not associated with aging, there is the probability of Alzheimer' disease. People with Alzheimer's disease often have trouble remembering where they left their properties such as parked vehicles or remembering what they want to buy at the mall.

Forgetting common words

Alzheimer's patient may experience trouble remembering everyday common word such as a chair. This is quite different from short-term memory loss, it is a case where the patient forgets totally the names of common things in and around the house. They resort to using descriptive phrases instead of common name for objects. The speech and understanding may be hampered, and loss of mind may be imminent.

Difficulty in learning new things

People suffering from Alzheimer's disease may find it difficult to learn new things. They tend to have a shorter attention span and repeating questions. Organizing their thought and thinking logically will be difficult if not impossible; some victim may lose their mental processing skills and often forget to pay for items bought.

Difficulty in performing the simple everyday task

Missing route to familiar places and or taking a longer time than usual in performing an everyday simple task may be a pointer to Alzheimer's disease. The individual becomes agitated and often have a terrible sleep pattern; they become so slow in action and reaction. If these symptoms are not associated with aging, there are chances that the individual is suffering from Alzheimer's disease

Behavioral changes

Individuals suffering from Alzheimer's disease may lose interest, energy and hitherto spontaneity to life. They become irritated and easily provoked; in adverse cases, the victim may lose inhibition. That is why some victims of Alzheimer's disease may undress in public places without the feeling of Inhibition. They may become paranoid and lose the ability to judge time and space, this will reflect in their behavioral changes as they tend to do things in the wrong places or time.

CHAPTER TWO

How to diagnose Alzheimer's disease

Diagnosing Alzheimer's disease early enough remain the greatest way of managing the disease. Physical diagnosis of Alzheimer's diseases involves evaluating the changes in cognitive and personality traits. Further evaluation of symptoms pointing to various stages of Alzheimer's disease progression will help to properly place the victim. It is very pertinent to note here that some cognitive changes experienced by Alzheimer's patients can also be a result of aging, therefore, it is of utmost importance to put age into consideration when evaluating an individual.

Evaluating Changes in Cognition

Disruptive memory loss

Short-term memory loss causes a disruptive or distorted attention. The victim will have troubles recounting information correctly after some time lapse. To evaluate a victim of memory loss tries telling them a story or a piece of information, ask them to recount what you told them some moments later. If they can't remember or tell it correctly, repeat the same line of test with some other information. If it comes out that they fail to recount the information and they exhibit other symptoms of Alzheimer's diseases, take them for a Doctor's evaluation. The may be chances they are suffering from Alzheimer's diseases.

The tendency to misplace things.

 Because e of poor judgment of time and places, People with Alzheimer's diseases often leave their belongings in strange places and have difficulty retracing their steps. They may be objects or belongings they do not use often, as time goes by the misplacement will extend to every object or belongings they use. Sometimes people with Alzheimer's may accuse others of misplacement of their belongings because they have difficulty remembering where and when they actually used the object.

To check if your loved one is exhibiting this symptom of Alzheimer's diseases, look out for a common object that is indispensable to the victim. Locate where he or she kept it, go him and ask him there whereabouts of the object. If he gets it correctly, try moving the object from where he kept it. This will give you the assurance that he has no tendency of misplacing things

Notice challenges in problem-solving.

 Understanding complex and multi-steps issues are particularly difficult for Alzheimer's patient. This may be linked to the disruptive or temporary memory loss. Working with numbers, solving complex problems and or basic mathematics may become difficult at the onset of Alzheimer's diseases. A person suffering from Alzheimer's diseases may find it difficult to follow a plan or follow complex road network. Try to ask your patient some simple arithmetic or the way to a particular store to see if he can solve it correctly. If you are in a car with them, ask them how to get to a local grocery or drug store

Look for confusion with time or place.

Many people suffering from Alzheimer's disease may have confusion with time, date and place. A simple doormat may appear to be a deep rectangular hole to them because of the failure of their brain to interpret space, time and distance correctly. Try asking him what date time and month is it. Place a doormat at the door to see if he will cross it.

Listen for speech problems.

 In advance case, people with Alzheimer's may lose track

of a conversation they're having or struggle to follow along. They may also mangle common words or phrases or repeat themselves. Watch out for slurring, using incorrect words, or random, strange pauses in conversation.

Give them a series of relatively long words with many syllables that you would expect them to know like "magnanimous," "unencumbered," and "perfidiousness" and ask them to repeat them back. If they slur or are unable to pronounce the word, this may be a sign of Alzheimer's.

Seek a medical evaluation.

When the aforementioned evaluation points to the way of Alzheimer's disease, it is best to take a medical evaluation from a physician to know the stage of the diseases. A mini-mental Status Examination will help to assess mental functions and neuropsychiatric testing. With the advancement in neuroimaging, the cognitive functions of the patient can be evaluated, the mini-mental status test will determine if the patient has abnormal or normal cognition. It will also determine if the patient is suffering from dementia or delirium.

The mental status examination evaluates patient on a scale of 1 to 30, an examination result of less than 24 out of 30 is considered a sign of cognitive deficiency. The mental evaluation will check for problems with arousal, concentration, memory, language, visual perception, executive functioning, mood, thoughts, praxis, and calculations of the patient.

Changes in Personality

As the mental condition of Alzheimer's patient worsens, it tends to put a heavy toll on their personality, there will be a considerable change in their social interactions and mood.

Social withdrawal.

 People with Alzheimer's often lose interest in social life such as their hobbies and work. This may be caused by the difficulties in recalling their last encounter with such activity. This, in addition, makes everything look strange and cumbersome; remember that Alzheimer's patient may find it difficult to cope with a complex problem such as relearning. They will rather withdraw from social life than to face strange and complex environment. When you observe a noticeable loss of interest in a hitherto interesting hobby, work and or friends you may go see a physician for proper evaluation.

Watch for changes in mood.

Confusion arising from short memory loss may cause an Alzheimer's patient to swing mood often. Look out for expressions that depict confusion, anger, frustration and or anxiety. Pay particular attention to how they behave when they are around new people or outside their comfort zone.

Look for poor judgment.

People with Alzheimer's often show poor judgment and decision-making ability. This will reflect in the dressing, eating and every sphere of their lives. Some Alzheimer's patient is known to put on their shoes wrongly, some may tend to wear their shirt inside out. As a result of disruptive memory, some Alzheimer's patient tends to trust and spend their money unwisely. There was a report of an Alzheimer's patient found with about sixteen credit cards from a financial institution, this clearly depicts how they can be easily deceived by an advert from salesmen or TV.

Identifying the Stages of Alzheimer's diseases

Onset stages.

The onset stages or early stages of Alzheimer's diseases may be very difficult to detect, there may be a decline in cognitive abilities which can be traceable to several other factors. Having a CTE scan of the brain will be the best way of detecting Alzheimer's disease at the early stage. Some symptoms of the early stage of Alzheimer's diseases are short-term memory loss, forgetting common names of objects, fumbling while talking and confusion.

Mid stages.

 The mid-stage of Alzheimer's diseases has a more pronounce symptom and last longer than the onset stages. Patient or sufferers begin to show odd behavior, loss of sense of hygiene and occasional relapse into long-term memory loss. The sufferer may need the assistance of caregivers to cope with everyday living because at this stage most sufferers may lose control of the bladder and may pass urine and pooh improperly.

Severe stages.

The last stage of Alzheimer's diseases is the severe stage, patients suffer long-term memory loss and inabilities to recall the past even their close relative and loved ones. Sufferers lose control of virtually all aspect of their lives and have to live on assistance from people. They may lose their ability to walk, talk or swallow food. The patient will need a round the clock monitoring preferably a home caregiver who is knowledgeable in managing people living with Alzheimer's diseases.

CHAPTER THREE

Reducing the risk of Alzheimer's diseases

At the moment, the scientist are working on finding a permanent cure for Alzheimer's diseases, therefore, preventing or reducing the risk of Alzheimer's diseases is very crucial. There are several ways to prevent or reduce the risk of Alzheimer's diseases by controlling the health-related risk through exercise, healthy lifestyle and others.

Controlling Health-Related Risk Factors

Regular Exercise.

Regular exercise probably 2 to 3 times a week help improves blood circulation to the brain and keep thinking and memory skills intact. Regular exercise is known to be a good regulator of blood pressure and cholesterol which are a major culprit in Alzheimer's diseases. Take a brisk walk for about 30 to 40 minutes 3 times a week or go swimming. It is particularly important to engage in the combination of cardiovascular exercise and strength training to build your muscles.

Maintain a brain-healthy diet.

To reduce the risk of Alzheimer's diseases, there is need to eat a diet that can stimulate a healthy brain. You may consider green vegetables, red wine, almond, blueberries, whole grain foods, fish, poultry and other healthy food capable of improving the memory. You must avoid some foods that are capable of shooting up your blood glucose or cholesterol levels such as red meat, cheese, margarine, pastries, and sugar. It is particularly important to consume a considerable amount of fish because they contain omega-3s, which are great for brain health. There are other foods that are high on omega 3s such as chia and flax seed but consuming a sizeable amount of fish 2 to 3 times a week may reduce your risk of Alzheimer's diseases by 60%

Monitor your Blood pressure and cholesterol level closely.

 High blood pressure and high cholesterol level have been severally linked to Alzheimer's diseases. Therefore, a close watch on your blood pressure and cholesterol level is very crucial in reducing the risk of Alzheimer's diseases. There is no lower limit of cholesterol level, therefore, the lower the better, but it must be kept within the limit of 100 mg/dl. An ideal blood pressure is 120/80, but this may vary with age and medical condition and it must not exceed 130/90. Problem with high blood pressure and high cholesterol level impact negatively on the brain and much pressure is mounted on the fragile veins in the brain, therefore it will increase the risk of Alzheimer's diseases.

To help regulate your blood pressure and cholesterol level cut down on table salt intake, leave processed foods out of your diet eat vegetables and fresh fruits instead.

Monitor your blood sugar.

Insulin failure or high intake of sugary products can result in high blood glucose know as diabetes. Diabetes is a silent killer disease because it has been linked severally to major renal and cardiovascular diseases. Every organ in the body has it a limit of sugar requirement, when there is excess glucose in the body and the insulin is enough to remove them from the blood, it is pushed to these major organs in the body including the heart kidney and brain. This has been the major cause of heart and kidney failure, also because of excess supply of sugar to the brain it may impact the brain negatively and increase the risk of Alzheimer's diseases. Ensure that your blood glucose is within the range of 70 to 99 mg/dl. Visit your physician regularly for routine check and advice on managing your blood glucose.

Quit smoking.

Studies show that smoking is one of the greatest risk factors for Alzheimer's diseases. Smokers above 65 years of age have about 80% higher risk than non-smokers. Quitting Smoking is one of the easiest ways to reduce the risk of Alzheimer's diseases because the soot, nicotine from smoking affect the brain negatively and increase the risk of Alzheimer's diseases.

Building a Brain-Healthy Lifestyle

Avoid head injury.

Head injury poses a great threat to healthy living, it is particularly true because having head injury increases the chances of one coming down on Alzheimer's diseases. Head injury can occur in an auto crash, fall, or during sport. It is very important to ensure safety and adequate protection of your head from injury while involving in any of these activities. In homes, cares should be taken to avoid falling down, never leave loose mats or slippery objects on the floor. If there are elderly people living with you, install handrail on stairways and every other places that may require supports while climbing.

Learn new skills.

Learn a new skill to keep your brain active and mentally fit. Join an adult class or lean a new game to challenge your brain and improve your mental health

Maintain active work life.

Maintaining your role in the workforce or business may help you stay sociable and active. Retiring too early from the workforce or business life may reduce your activity that may encourage your health to deteriorate. Remaining in your job keeps you mentally and physically active and fit, this will have a positive effect on your mental health.

Maintain a good Sleep pattern.

To maintain a healthy lifestyle, it is required for everyone to have at least 7 to 8 hours of sleep each day. Insufficient sleep on a long run will reduce your efficiency and pose adverse effects on your mental wellbeing. If you suspect sleep apnea, get medical assistance from your physician so that you can get adequate sleep.

Avoid unnecessary stress.

Stress impact your life negatively, it stimulates the release of some hormone in your body that will impact it negatively. Also, stress can shoot up your blood pressure which is a link to Alzheimer's diseases. Avoiding stress or reducing your stress level can keep your brain healthy and active. Find a way to engage in activities that help calm your nerves down. Consider taking a walk in the park or doing yoga, take a warm bath or go to the beach to relax.

Learn how to manage and respond to stress if your job or another aspect of your life gives you stress, train your brain to tackle stress in a positive a manner in order to reduce the effects on you.

Taking Vitamins and Medications

Take vitamin E daily.

Taking about 5mg of vitamin E daily help to improve your health. Vitamin E is an antioxidant that helps to fights free radicals in the body. Free radicals are very dangerous in the body causing damages to body cells and organs including the brain. Vitamin E is abundant in mangos paw-paw, tomatoes, red pepper, and spinach. Consuming a sizable amount of these edibles on daily basis will help supply your body with the needed amount of vitamin E.

Take vitamin B and folate supplements.

Vitamin B and folate supplements are particularly helpful in preventing brain deterioration. Vitamin B9 is made up of folic acid, folic acid, when combined with vitamin B12, may help to slow down or prevent brain deterioration. Also, the use of Vitamin D, magnesium and fish oil will give additional remedies to a brain problem

There several foods that contain these vitamins such as lentils, spinach, beets, and broccoli. Also, cauliflower, parsley, collard green and romaine lettuce contains these vitamins, supplementing your diet with them will help supply them to your brain

vitamin B12 and other B vitamins can be found in fishes, potatoes, eggs, poultry, cereal. red meat can also be a good source of such vitamins but be very moderate when eating red meat because it is linked with cholesterol.

Consider the use of Berberine.

Berberine was used in ancient medicine, it is noted for its capability to lower blood pressure and cholesterol level. It is made up of extracts from Barberry, Oregon grape, Chinese Goldthread and Goldenseal. There are ongoing researches about its possible use in the treatment of diseases, talk to your physician about using berberine as herbal supplements

Look into Alpha-GPC.

 Alpha-GPC combines with other medication can help in delaying or slowing down the progression of Alzheimer's diseases. Alpha-GPC is generally considered as safe medication in many countries across the world, talk to your physician about the possible combination of Alpha-GPC with your drugs.

Follow your doctor's prescription.

 There are classes of drugs used in managing Alzheimer's disease, follow the prescription of your doctor. Never fail to consult your doctor when in doubt or noticing some abnormal reactions from the drugs. Drugs such as cholinesterase inhibitors may help in improving a mild case of Alzheimer's or Dementia. Aricept, Exelon, and Razadyne are also good in treating Alzheimer's diseases but must not be taken without a doctor's prescription.

CHAPTER FOUR

How to treat Alzheimer's diseases

Treating Alzheimer's disease may be very tasking because there is no cure at the moments. Scientists are trying their best in research institution to find a cure for the Alzheimer's diseases, therefore the available drugs are meant to slow down or treat some of the symptoms of the disease. Alzheimer's disease affects the brain of it sufferers causing a deterioration and gradual loss of memory. Treating Alzheimer's diseases entails creating a support for sufferers, safe environment, and coping strategies.

Medications options

Collaborate with your doctor for a treatment plan.

 If you are diagnosed with Alzheimer's disease, talk with your doctor about the possible treatment plan with respect to your case. There are several medication options that you can choose from with the help of your physician, this must be done after due consideration of your overall health condition, the stage of the disease and its associated symptoms.

Try talking to your doctor about your fears of future symptoms, and the side effects of the chosen drugs.

Consider cholinesterase inhibitors to Improve cognitive function.

Cholinesterase inhibitors such as galantamine and rivastigmine are good in improving the brain function in the early stage of Alzheimer's diseases. It is also called AChE Inhibitors used by many people in slowing down the progression of brain damage and memory loss. Although these drugs are great for managing Alzheimer's disease they come with a side effect, therefore it must not be taken without the advice of your doctor.

Memantine is good to manage more severe Alzheimer's symptoms.

Memantine also called Namenda is good in treating Alzheimer's diseases. It comes in pills and capsules, it helps to slow down the progression of Alzheimer's diseases in the later stage. Memenda can interact with other supplements such as vitamins used in the treatment of Alzheimer's diseases. Memantine must not be taken with the approval of a competent medical personnel or your doctor.

Managing a Safe and Supportive Environment for Alzheimer's patient

Join a support group.

Managing Alzheimer's disease is becomes easier with support from people around you. Join a support group in your area or online where people who are sufferers or caregivers share their experience with the diseases. This will help in giving you some support and information that you will need to manage your condition. Talk to your family member and friends about your condition and tell them how they may help you in coping with the diseases.

Consider the help of a caregiver.

Caregivers are people that can give you support in daily living with Alzheimer's diseases, they may come for few hours of the day or live with you to provide daily support for you. This is very important especially in the severe stage when the patient is suffering from long-term memory loss and may not be able to walk or eat without a third party support. Talk with your doctor and insurance company on the best caregiver option you will need to cope with the diseases.

Create an environment for easy movement around

your home.

Try and create a good arrangement for your home to help you move around easily without obstructions. Due to a problem with coordination, people suffering from Alzheimer's disease may find it difficult to move around therefore improper placement of object around the house create an additional problem for them. Ensure to keep lose carpet out of the floor, fix lose rail grabbings and slippery spots in the house. Remove unused furniture and clutters from the house to help create a coping system for the Alzheimer's patients

Fix handrails in difficult areas of the home.

Stairways and bathrooms may be particularly difficult for Alzheimer's patient. They may fall while trying to climb the stairs or washing their feet in the bathroom if there are no hand supports, therefore, it may be necessary to install handrails and support in the bathrooms, stairways and other difficult areas of the house to give them support in moving around the house

Create a diary.

Having a diary is one sure way to manage long-term memory loss. Create a diary that may contain the names and phone numbers of people you always contact such as your doctor or caregiver, you can also create an album of the photograph of your favorite people and places to help you with a sense of comfort and stability.

Creating a Coping Approach

Enlist an occupational therapist.

Get an occupational therapist to help you deal with some difficult task such as taking medications and meals. Ask them to help you develop a feasible coping strategy with reference to your case and symptoms.

Get advice from your insurance company and your healthcare provider when considering the service of an occupational therapist.

Get a cognitive therapist.

A cognitive therapist may help you to manage and build strategies to improve your thinking skills. A combination of cognitive therapy and medication may be very effective in managing people living with Alzheimer's diseases. They design approaches and ways to help engage your mind to help improve your memory, thinking skills, and emotional balances. There is a cognitive behavioral therapist (CBT) and cognitive stimulation therapist (CST), talk with your doctor about the best option for your condition

Talk to a psychologist.

Talking with a psychologist is a wonderful way of managing some symptoms associated with Alzheimer's disease. You will get help on how to manage depression, anxiety, and irritation that comes with Alzheimer's diseases. You may also involve in arts such as music to improve your memory and brain functions

Regular exercise is very important.

Going for regular exercise help to improve your mood, it also stimulates blood flow in the brain. Decide on the best exercise for you, talk to your doctor so that he can advise you on the best way to do exercise from your health point of view. There are some very basic exercises such as walking, bicycling and dancing that are safe for almost every health conditions. You can decide on one of them and talk to your healthcare provider about it.

Set reminder alarms and calendars.

Set alarms to remind you of important appointment such as seeing your doctor or taking your medications. Mark important dates out on your calendar and add little notes to the dates to help you remember and understand the nature of the appointment.

CHAPTER FIVE

Caring for Alzheimer's patient

Caring for an Alzheimer's diseases patient is a daunting task especially at the severe stage of the diseases when the patient needs around the clock care and monitoring. At the onset stage, the patient may still be able to do some basic things such as walking, eating, and cleaning. But as the diseases progress, the patient may have long-term memory loss resulting from deteriorating brain, therefore he may lose his ability to coordinate himself. He may lose his ability to swallow food or remember faces, he may exhibit some abnormal characters such as incoherent murmuring, improper dressing or going naked. Therefore a third party caregiver is very crucial to help the patient cope. A caregiver could be anybody from close relatives or hired professional caregivers who must be available to the patient for support. Caregiving involves creating a safe environment for sufferers, helping in creating a good coping strategy and providing health and wellbeing support.

Health Care and well-being support.

Liaise with healthcare provider.

A caregiver for Alzheimer's patient should be able to liaise with a healthcare provider to keep the patient healthy at all times. It is very important for the caregiver to have some basic knowledge of the disease in order to understand and provide the right support for the patient. Caregiver must be able to work out modalities with the assistance of doctors, nurses, case managers and other social workers to provide important information that will help tailor a strategy that may be effective in slowing down the progression of the diseases.

A caregiver is a link bridge between the patient and the health professionals, he must provide information of any changes to the health personnel in charge of the case promptly in order to reduce the frustration of the patient.

Obtain the patient permission to care for him.

Obtain permission from the patient or a consensus agreement in the case of a family member such as parents. The permission allows you to take decisions promptly and provide adequate help for the patient. There are several cases of siblings fighting over the custody of their parents; this must be well iron out from inception because disagreement like that can hamper the progression in providing adequate care for the patient.

When seeking legal consent from your patient, speak in clear and audible voice, target a stable time for your patient to speak to him. Ensure he understands what you want from him, give him room for questioning so that you will be sure there is no ambiguity in your request and action.

Give proper attention to medications.

Proper medication is very important in slowing down the progression of Alzheimer's diseases, therefore caregiver must ensure that the patient takes his daily prescription as at when due. It is also the responsibility of the caregiver to get a refill of medications that have been used. Caregiver must see to it that the patient gets an appropriate daily dose of sleep, inform the healthcare professionals in the case of anxiety and poor sleep pattern.

Understand the dosing instructions for every medication of your patient. Keep a record of medications to ensure the person takes the daily doses. Pay attention to the times the person takes the medication and any complications. Provide this information to the healthcare personnel as at when due to help them provide adequate medical advice for the patient.

Study some common Alzheimer's medications and treatments.

Learn some common Alzheimer's medications such as Memantine, an N-methyl-D-aspartate that slow down the process that breaks down the important neurotransmitters of the brain. Read more about some common symptoms of Alzheimer's diseases and the common treatment for them such as zolpidem for sleep medication and lorazepam for anxiety disorder.

Create a regular routine for a checkup.

Creating a regular medical check-up routine, help make the patient accessible for medical examination and monitoring. Scheduling a routine medical check-up to support the patient sense of well-being, talk to the healthcare provider about the need and possibility of a routine medical examination in order to to be proactive about the progress of the diseases.

Managing Frustrations

Identify the source of frustration.

You cannot isolate frustration from Alzheimer's disease. People suffering from Alzheimer's diseases may be frustrated, agitated and irritated as a result of complications from the deterioration of the brain. Caregivers must figure out the source of their frustrations and help to create easier steps for the routine. The caregiver may have the buttons replaced with a zipper or snaps if doing the buttons is becoming frustrating. At restaurants and public gatherings, the caregiver must ensure a comfortable and safe place for the patient; help him to select menu or less complex seats at the gathering.

Manage a necessary routine.

 Caregiver must figure out ways to manage a necessary routine such as eating, cleaning, and dressing. Create an easy schedule and routine for the patient to learn. Make the routine less complex in order to help the patient reduce the frustrations associated with learning a new routine. Do not rush the patient while teaching him a new routine, give room for relaxation so that he will not lose interest in the entire process. In the case of routine outside the house or that required additional preparation such as seeing a doctor, start preparing the patient ahead of time to give him adequate time to get dressed or wash.

Involve your patient in some task.

Allow your patient to take up some task such as dressing up independently, this will help boost his wellbeing and stimulate the proper blood flow in the brain. Ensure that the task is very simple and less demanding because demanding tasks can wear him out.

Make instructions simple.

Giving instructions is inevitable in managing Alzheimer's patient. Caregivers must ensure that the instructions are very simple and clear, this is to avert confusion and frustrations. If a patient finds it difficult to understand instructions from caregivers, they may be Confused and frustrated, ensure that you have your patient's attention when giving the instruction, cross check to be sure the patient understand your instructions.

Creating a Safe Environment

How to prevent fall.

For Alzheimer's patient, fall may be rampant if proper care is not taken. Their deteriorating mental condition impairs their coordination abilities and reduces stability; therefore, necessary precaution must be put in place to prevent them from falling down. Keep all clutter and dirt capable of causing a slip or tilt from the patient ways, avoid the use of loose rugs and doormats that is capable of causing a slip for the patient. Extension wires and cables are very dangerous for people living with Alzheimer's disease because it can cause a great fall and injury to the head which may worsen the patient condition.

Install handrails at the stairways and bathrooms to give them support at difficult areas of the house.

Use locks as security measures.

In severe stage of Alzheimer's disease, the patient may wander away from home or get injured by harmful materials; therefore, it is very important to install locks on doors and cabinet that contains potentially hazardous materials. If your patient has a history of wandering away from home, install safety lock on all your doors high enough so that he cannot unlock them and go out. Places containing alcohol, medicine, weapons, and chemical must be kept under lock and key at all times to prevent your patient from entering there and harming himself.

Control water temperatures.

Alzheimer's patient has a problem with judgment, they may not be able to regulate water heater properly. If they are left without supervision, they may sustain injuries from hot water. Therefore water heater must be adequately monitored, it is an extra precaution to install water temperature controller at bath and kitchen sinks to help prevent burns from hot water.

Keep lighters and flammables out of reach.

Alzheimer's patient may have confusion with matches and lighters; this may be very dangerous if there are flammable materials around. Alzheimer's caregiver must ensure that lighters and flammable materials are kept out of the reach of the patient at all times to prevent fire burns and injuries. Install fire extinguishers and smoke detectors in your home, in the case of a smoker which is highly discouraged, supervise every session of smoking and ensure that all flames and fires are put out at the end of the session.

Create a safe place for valuables.

People living with Alzheimer's disease often have a problem with location, they can misplace valuable materials and can never retrace their locations, therefore its very important to keep valuables such as keys, wallets and other important materials in the house from the reach of the patient. Create a safe rack and ensure that the patient keeps his valuables on the rack so that he can easily locate them when needed.

Manage to wander appropriately.

In the case of Alzheimer's diseases, wandering may be inevitable; the patient may wander away from home or miss his route and go missing. The memory loss associated with Alzheimer's disease cause the patient to forget his route thereby wandering about the house or neighborhood. Caregiver must take note of the history of wandering, try and figure out the nature of the wandering so as to know the cause of the wandering. A patient who wanders every morning may be suffering from hunger, therefore caregiver must ensure to provide food early enough for such patient to help solve the case of wandering.

In an extreme case, caregivers must ensure that the patient wears a name tag containing contact information so that you can be contacted in the case of missing way.

Keep mirrors and other injurious materials away.

A person suffering from Alzheimer's disease may lose his memory, seeing his image on mirror may be very frightening; therefore keep all mirrors at bay. If the use of a mirror is inevitable, ensure to supervise it and keep it away after use. Also, other mirrors that have no other use other than cosmetic for the house should be kept away to help the patient reduce anxiety and frustrations.

www.ingramcontent.com/pod-product-compliance
Lightning Source LLC
Chambersburg PA
CBHW070100260726
48658CB00002B/923